Pregnancy 101 for Dads

Everything You Need to Know About Pregnancy and Beyond

DR. ELVIRA S. GRAVES

TABLE OF CONTENTS

Disclaimer

Introduction

Greetings from the exciting and life-changing world of fatherhood! You're about to set out on an experience unlike any other, whether you're feeling excited, nervous, or a combination of all three. Special pleasures, difficulties, and obligations are associated with being an expecting father. This introduction is meant to be the first step toward accepting this responsibility with assurance, comprehension, and a feeling of direction. Let's get started.

Being a father involves a deep commitment to loving, caring for, and guiding your child; it's more than just a title. This path is filled with innumerable opportunities for development, education, and life-changing events. Every stage, from the time you find out you are pregnant until the baby's birth and beyond, has its advantages and disadvantages. With the information and resources you need to be the greatest father you can be, this handbook is here to help you every step of the way.

Although the path ahead may appear difficult, it will also be immensely fulfilling. Consider it a marathon instead of a race. At times, you may experience feelings of overload, uncertainty, or even fear. That is quite typical. The secret is to go into this adventure with an open mind and a desire to learn. Accept the uncertainty, treasure the happy times, and be ready for anything. Keep in mind that you are not alone in this. This journey has been traveled by millions of fathers before you, and many are currently treading it with you.

One of the first things you'll discover is that pregnancy is an emotional adventure for both of you, not just your partner. You will see directly the amazing physical and emotional transformations your companion experiences. Being there for her, providing patience, understanding, and support, is crucial. This is your path as well as hers. You're already beginning the process of becoming a wonderful father by being actively involved.

It's critical to understand how significant your support and involvement are as you get ready to accept the role of an expectant father. According to studies, men who are actively involved in their children's lives during pregnancy and delivery typically develop closer bonds with them and have more positive relationships with their partners. There is more to your duty than merely watching. You play a crucial role in this process, and your presence, words, and deeds can have a big impact.

Learning more about pregnancy and childbirth is one way to get involved. Knowledge is power, and the more you comprehend the situation, the more capable you will be of managing any obstacles that may come along. Spend some time learning about your partner's changes, the various phases of pregnancy, and what to anticipate throughout labor and delivery. Read books, go to prenatal classes, and don't be afraid to ask questions. Your level of confidence will increase with your level of knowledge.

Another essential component of being a supportive partner is communication. Your spouse may go through mood swings, worry, and anxiety throughout pregnancy, which can be a roller coaster of emotions. It
is crucial to establish a welcoming and encouraging atmosphere where she can freely express her emotions. Be patient, reassure, and actively listen. Keep in mind that you are a team, and cooperating will improve your relationship and make this journey easier for you.

Apart from providing emotional support, there are also useful techniques to prepare for your child's birth. First, assemble the necessities and set up the nursery. This includes items like diapers, baby clothes, a changing table, and a cot. Along with talking about your preferences and expectations for labor and delivery, it's a good idea to draft a birth plan. This can guarantee that you are both on the same page and help reduce some of the anxiousness.

Another crucial factor to take into account is financial preparation. There are costs associated with raising a child, so planning is essential. Review your finances, make a budget, and begin saving for the future of your child. This could entail prioritizing your financial objectives and changing your spending patterns. You may give your expanding family a stable and safe environment by taking proactive measures.

You'll find helpful hints, professional counsel, and first-hand accounts from other fathers who have been in your position as you go through this guide. From comprehending the fundamentals of pregnancy to being ready for the baby's arrival and beyond, each chapter is made to give you the

knowledge you require. With its abundance of information, encouragement, and support, this guide is designed to be your traveling companion.

Keep in mind that no father is flawless. It's acceptable to make mistakes. Your readiness to develop, learn, and support your partner and child is what counts. Being a father is a lifelong learning process that is full of highs and lows, tears and laughter, and victories and failures. Enjoy every second, treasure the memories, and know that you're doing a fantastic job.

Therefore, know that you're making a significant step toward becoming the best father you can be, regardless of whether you read this guide from beginning to end or use it as a guide along the road. This is your adventure, your journey, and your chance to positively influence your child's life. Greetings from fatherhood. Let's begin!

Chapter 1: Fundamentals of Pregnancy

Pregnancy is a unique experience that involves poignant moments and major changes. For both you and your partner, it's a period of change and development. Knowing the fundamentals of pregnancy will help you, as an expectant father, go through this time more easily and confidently. The basic elements of pregnancy, such as the trimesters, significant life events, typical symptoms, and the vital role of prenatal care, will be covered in this chapter. Usually, a pregnancy lasts three trimesters, each lasting roughly three months. Every trimester has its own unique experiences, difficulties, and developments.

Weeks 112 of the First Trimester

Conception marks the start of the first trimester, which ends after the 12th week. The fertilized egg attaches itself to the uterine lining during this period, and the embryo starts to grow. By the end of this trimester, the embryo has developed into a fetus, and the baby's main organs and systems have begun to take shape. Your companion may have major changes and symptoms at this time.

Your spouse may have mood changes, morning sickness, exhaustion, and frequent urination. Although these symptoms can be difficult, they are a typical aspect of the first trimester of pregnancy. Being empathetic and encouraging during this time is crucial. Encourage your significant other to take breaks, eat small, frequent meals, and drink plenty of water. Despite its name, morning sickness can strike at any time of day. Crackers or ginger tea could help ease some of the pain.

During the first trimester, emotional changes are also typical. Feelings of joy or anxiety as well as mood swings can result from the hormonal changes. Listening patiently and sympathetically can have a big impact. Assure your significant other that these emotions are typical and that you will be there for her no matter what.

Weeks 1326 of the Second Trimester

Pregnancy's second trimester is frequently regarded as the most pleasurable. Your companion may start feeling more energized as many of the initial symptoms, such as weariness and nausea, start to go away. You might even feel the baby move for the first time at this point, and you'll probably notice your partner's growing baby bump.

The baby continues to grow and develop quickly throughout this trimester. The baby's motions become more apparent as the organs that developed during the first trimester begin to mature. Additionally, you will have the chance to view your unborn child via ultrasound at this time, which will be an exciting event for you both. Your partner can develop new symptoms like heartburn, leg cramps, and back pain. Helping her figure out how to get rid of these discomforts is crucial. Encourage her to engage in regular exercise, like yoga or walking, and make sure she eats a nutritious diet.

Additionally, now is an excellent time to begin getting ready for the baby's arrival. Important things to do include talking about your birth plan, setting up the nursery, and going to prenatal classes. Participating fully in these preparations will benefit your partner and improve your relationship.

The 2740th week of the third trimester

The last stage of the pregnancy is the third trimester. Your partner's body is preparing for labor and delivery, and the baby is still growing and gaining weight. Due to the baby's growing growth and increasingly noticeable symptoms, this trimester can be emotionally and physically taxing.

Your companion can have trouble breathing, have swollen ankles and feet, and have trouble sleeping. It's critical to offer empathy and support throughout this period. To lessen her tension, help her discover comfortable sleeping positions, promote frequent pauses and relaxation, and offer assistance with housework.

You will both need to be ready for labor and delivery as the due date draws near. Talk about your choices for labor and delivery, pack the hospital bag, and attend childbirth classes together. You can determine when it's time to visit the hospital by being aware of the symptoms of labor, including contractions and water breaking.

Typical Pregnancy Signs and How to Help Your Spouse

We've already discussed a few of the many symptoms that come with pregnancy. It's important to know what to anticipate and how to help your partner through these changes.

Morning Sickness: Your partner may experience nausea and vomiting. Encourage her to stay hydrated, eat small, frequent meals, and stay away from foods that make her feel queasy. Acupressure wristbands or ginger products might also be beneficial.

Fatigue: The first and third trimesters of pregnancy can be particularly taxing. Don't overburden your partner with work and make sure she gets enough sleep. To relieve her workload, offer to assist with errands and housework.

Back discomfort: Your partner's center of gravity may change as the baby grows, which may cause back discomfort. To ease her discomfort, encourage her to utilize supportive pillows, maintain proper posture, and think about doing mild exercises or pregnant yoga.

Heartburn: This condition might be brought on by hormonal fluctuations and the developing fetus. Encourage your companion to avoid fatty or spicy foods, eat smaller, more frequent meals, and stand up straight after eating. Although over-the-counter antacids might also help, it's preferable to speak with her doctor.

Mood Swings: Mood swings can result from hormonal changes. Offer consolation and support while listening with patience and empathy. Let your partner know that it's acceptable for her to express her feelings and promote open conversation.

Foot and ankle swelling is frequent, particularly during the third trimester. Encourage your significant other to drink plenty of water, avoid standing for extended periods, and raise her feet whenever she can. Swelling may also be lessened using compression stockings.

The Function of Prenatal Healthcare

An essential component of a healthy pregnancy is prenatal care. Seeing a doctor on a regular basis guarantees that the baby and your spouse are healthy and growing normally. These consultations offer a chance to track the baby's development, look for any possible issues, and answer any queries or worries you may have.

Your spouse will go through several tests and screenings during prenatal checkups to make sure everything is going according to plan. These could consist of ultrasounds, blood tests, and urine tests. The medical professional will also keep an eye on your partner's general health, blood pressure, and weight.

If at all possible, you should go with your partner to these appointments. Your attendance demonstrates your involvement and support throughout the pregnancy process. You can ask any questions you may have and find out more about the baby's development during this time. As an expectant father, you will feel more prepared and confident if you are informed and involved.

Making healthy lifestyle choices is another aspect of prenatal care. Encourage your significant other to consume a well-rounded diet full of lean proteins, healthy grains, fruits, and vegetables. Regular exercise, like swimming or walking, is another way to stay active. Make sure she gets enough sleep and stays away from drugs and alcohol that could affect the unborn child, such as certain medications.

Preparing for the emotional and psychological changes that accompany pregnancy is another crucial component of prenatal care. Your partner's mood and mental health may be affected by hormonal changes. Pay attention to what she needs emotionally and provide a sympathetic ear. She should be encouraged to speak with her healthcare physician if she is feeling severe stress, anxiety, or depression. During pregnancy, mental and physical wellness are equally crucial.

For both of you, prenatal classes are a great resource. From preparing for childbirth to caring for and nursing infants, these seminars cover a wide range of subjects. They offer useful knowledge and useful techniques that will boost your self-esteem and confidence as you get closer to giving birth.

It's crucial to talk to your healthcare professional about your birth plan as the due date draws near. Your choices for labor and delivery are detailed in a birth plan, together with information about who you want to be there, how you want pain to be managed, and any special requests you may have. Although flexibility is crucial, having a plan in place helps ease worry and guarantee that you and your partner agree.

Being a caring and involved expecting father begins with knowing the fundamentals of pregnancy. Every stage of pregnancy presents different difficulties and chances for development, from the early signs of the first trimester to the third trimester's labor and delivery preparations. You're setting the stage for a healthy pregnancy and a solid relationship with your spouse and unborn child by educating yourself, providing practical and emotional support, and taking part in prenatal care.

For both you and your partner, pregnancy is a transformative experience. Accept this period with an open mind and a desire to learn. In addition to helping you get through the months of pregnancy, the information and abilities you acquire will get you ready for the amazing experience that is fatherhood. Welcome to this incredible journey, and congrats on starting down the path to becoming a fantastic father.

Chapter 2: Getting Ready for the Infant

The process of getting ready for your baby's arrival may be both thrilling and daunting. There are a lot of things to think about, such as choosing the appropriate baby equipment, budgeting for new expenses, and setting up the nursery. This chapter will walk you through these crucial milestones, assisting you in making your home cozy and inviting for your child and making sure you're ready financially for the journey.

Getting the Nursery Ready

One of the most fun aspects of getting ready for your baby's arrival is designing a cozy and secure nursery. Playtime, those priceless first grins, and late-night feedings are just a few of the special times that will take place in the nursery. These are the necessities for creating a comfortable and useful nursery.

First, think about the room's arrangement. Select a location that is peaceful, convenient, and spacious enough to hold all of the required furnishings and infant supplies. To protect your infant, you should place the crib away from windows and electrical outlets. Blackout curtains can be used to help create a calming, dark space for nighttime and naps.

Mattress and Crib: The nursery's focal point is the crib. Verify that it has a firm, well-fitting mattress and complies with current safety regulations. To lower the risk of SIDS, stay away from using pillows, stuffed animals, or soft bedding in the crib. Your infant only needs a fitted sheet to sleep comfortably and safely.

Changing Table: Diaper changes can be made more convenient with a special changing table or a dresser with a changing pad on top. To avoid straining your back, make sure it is at a comfortable height and includes safety straps. For quick and simple access, keep diapering necessities like wipes, creams, and diapers close at hand.

Storage Options: Infants have a lot of belongings! Having enough storage is crucial for anything from toys and clothing to food and cosmetics. To keep everything organized, think about combining containers, drawers, and shelves. Finding what you need quickly can be facilitated by labeling storage containers.

Comfortable Seating: For feeding sessions and lulling your infant to sleep, a comfortable chair or glider is essential. Select a chair that supports your back well, and for longer periods, think about adding a little side table to carry supplies like water, burp cloths, and a book or tablet.

Lighting: In the nursery, soft, movable lighting is essential. A nightlight or dimmable bulb can provide a soothing environment without being too hard on your infant's eyes. Additionally, it facilitates diaper changes and nocturnal feedings without completely waking your infant.

Pleasant to Have in the Nursery

A few nice-to-have items might give your nursery more comfort and convenience, but the necessities will get you started.

Sound Machine: To help your infant fall asleep, a sound machine that plays nature sounds, lullabies, or white noise can block out home disturbances.

Humidifier: Keeping the right amount of humidity in your home will help your baby breathe easier and avoid dry skin, especially in the winter or other dry seasons.

Books and Toys: A modest selection of soft toys and baby books can entertain and encourage early growth. Make acceptable and safe selections.

Decor: Give your infant a happy, stimulating atmosphere by personalizing the nursery with wall art, mobiles, and other decorations that express your personal taste.

Financial Planning: Baby Budgeting

Having a baby involves not just physical and emotional changes, but also financial ones. Being financially ready will ease your stress and guarantee that you can support your infant's requirements without jeopardizing the financial security of your family.

Start with a Budget: The first step is to make a thorough budget that accounts for all possible costs related to giving birth. This covers medical expenses, infant supplies, clothing, diapers, and childcare if required.

Medical Costs: The costs of prenatal treatment, birth, and postpartum care can be high. To find out what is covered and any potential out-of-pocket expenses, speak with your health insurance carrier. Additionally, it's a good idea to save money for unforeseen medical costs.

Baby Equipment and Supplies: As was already noted, the initial cost of setting up the nursery and buying baby equipment might be high. Set priorities for necessities and search for ways to cut costs, including borrowing from friends and family or purchasing used goods. To prevent wasting money, make a list of necessities and follow it.

Continuous Expenses: Infants develop rapidly, and their requirements are ever-changing. Set aside money for recurring expenses like clothing, formula (if not nursing), diapers, and baby food. To obtain an accurate picture of your monthly spending, it is beneficial to monitor these costs over time.

Childcare: Take into account the cost of childcare if you or your spouse intend to go back to work after the baby is delivered. These expenses can mount up regardless of whether you go with a nanny, home care, or a daycare facility. To assist with these costs, start looking into your alternatives as soon as possible and think about opening a daycare savings account.

Parental Leave: Recognize your company's parental leave guidelines and make appropriate plans. While some companies provide paid leave, others do not. You can better organize your finances and make sure you have enough resources to cover any unpaid leave if you are aware of your leave alternatives.

Emergency Fund: Having an emergency fund can bring peace of mind while dealing with the increased obligations that come with having a kid. To cover unforeseen expenses or crises, try to save three to six months' worth of living expenses.

Baby Equipment and Devices: Essentials

It can be difficult to choose the best baby equipment and devices, but it's crucial to concentrate on what you need to keep your child safe and happy. Here is a list of things you should always have on hand.

Car Seat: Bringing your kid home from the hospital and on all subsequent trips requires a car seat that is both safe and correctly placed. Verify that the car seat is suitable for your baby's age and size and satisfies current safety regulations. To make sure it's done right, think about having a qualified expert install it.

Stroller: A quality stroller may enhance the convenience and enjoyment of your baby's outings. Choose one that is stable, manageable, and able to develop with your child. Certain strollers have characteristics like plenty of storage space, grips that can be adjusted, and compatibility with car seats.

Baby Carrier: With a baby carrier, you can hold your infant close while freeing up your hands. Select one that is adjustable for a comfortable fit and provides good support for both you and your child.

Diapers & Wipes: Since you'll use them up rapidly, stock up on these items. Make sure you have enough diapers to last a few days and have a plan for refilling them, regardless of whether you decide to use cloth or disposable ones.

Feeding Supplies: Get some nursing bras and a cozy nursing cushion if your companion is nursing. Bottles, nipples, formula (if not nursing), and a bottle brush are required for bottle feeding.

Clothing: Keep a variety of onesies, sleepers, and clothes in different sizes because babies grow up quickly. Select materials that are easy to put on and take off, soft, and breathable. Remember to pack necessities like mittens, hats, and socks.

Bedding: You'll need a few swaddle blankets and fitted crib sheets in addition to a crib and mattress. For safety, keep heavy pillows and blankets out of the crib.

Bathing Supplies: The necessities for bath time are a baby bathtub, mild baby soap, shampoo, and soft towels. Never leave your infant alone in the bathtub, and make sure the water is at a suitable temperature.

First Aid Kit: A well-stocked first aid kit should have basic equipment like nail clippers, a digital thermometer, a nasal aspirator, and baby-safe drugs. Keeping a baby care manual and emergency contact information handy is also a smart idea.

Optional Devices: Some devices can help with parenting, but they are not required.

Baby Monitor: By enabling you to see your child even while you're not in the same room, a baby monitor can provide you peace of mind. If you'd like, pick one with video capability, crisp audio, and a reasonable range.

Bottle Warmer: By rapidly heating formula or breast milk to the proper temperature, a bottle warmer can help you save time and effort when feeding at night.

Swing or Bouncer: When you need some alone time, a baby swing or bouncer might come in quite handy. These gadgets use vibrations or soft rocking to help calm your infant.

Pacifiers: For certain infants, pacifiers provide comfort. Keeping a few on hand can help calm your fussy infant.

High Chair: A high chair is necessary as soon as your infant begins eating solid foods. Choose one that can be modified as your baby develops, has a secure harness, and is simple to clean.

Getting ready for the birth of your child requires careful preparation and thought. You may guarantee a seamless transition into parenting by organizing a cozy and secure nursery, planning for future financial adjustments, and selecting the appropriate baby supplies. Keep in mind that the most crucial thing is to provide your infant with a kind and encouraging atmosphere. Accept the journey and savor the priceless moments that occur along the route. Greetings from the wonderful world of parenthood!

Chapter 3: Health and Wellness

Maintaining one's health and well-being throughout pregnancy is of the utmost importance for both the mother-to-be and the developing child. The role that you play in providing support to your spouse during this moment of transition is extremely important if you are an expectant father. This chapter discusses the most important components of physical health and emotional well-being, as well as the significance of maintaining a healthy diet and engaging in physical activity while pregnant.

Making sure that your partner is taking care of their physical health is one of the most important things you can do for them. A woman's body is subjected to great demands throughout pregnancy, and the assistance that you provide can make a significant difference.

Participating in and keeping abreast of the situation is one of the most effective strategies to promote her physical health. Gain an understanding of the changes that are occurring in her body and the things that she needs throughout this period. For instance, knowing that weariness is a typical occurrence, particularly throughout the first and third trimesters of pregnancy, might assist you in being more compassionate and sympathetic. When she needs rest and naps, encourage her to take them.

To alleviate some of the stress that she is experiencing, you can assist her by taking over some of the responsibilities around the house.

Physical comfort is another area where your support might be useful. As her body changes, she may endure discomfort including back aches, swollen feet, and difficulties sleeping. You can help by delivering back massages, helping her find comfortable sleeping positions, and recommending strategies to reduce edema, such as elevating her feet or using compression stockings.

Encouraging regular prenatal checkups is also vital. These sessions are crucial for monitoring the health of both your partner and the baby. Go with her to these appointments whenever feasible. It shows your support and allows you both a chance to ask questions and stay informed about the pregnancy's progress.

Emotional well-being is as crucial throughout pregnancy. Hormonal fluctuations can lead to mood swings and emotional ups and downs. Your companion could feel pleased one moment and overwhelmed the next. Understanding these changes and being there for her emotionally can make a tremendous difference.

One effective technique to assist her mental well-being is through active listening. When she shares her feelings, listens without judgment and shows empathy. Sometimes, all she needs is someone to listen to and validate her feelings. For instance, if she expresses dread about the approaching birth, acknowledge her concerns and reassure her that it's natural to feel that way. You might also recommend practical ways to prepare for the delivery, such as taking childbirth classes together.

Reducing stress is another crucial part of emotional well-being. Help her discover methods to relax and unwind. This could include activities like taking a stroll together, enjoying a pregnant yoga class, or simply having a quiet evening at home. Be sensitive to her emotional needs and offer support in ways that are significant to her.

Encouraging open communication is crucial. Make it apparent that she can chat with you about anything that's on her mind. Whether it's her dreams and worries or just her daily experiences, being a supportive and understanding spouse helps develop a deep emotional connection.

Nutrition and exercise play a crucial part in maintaining health and fitness during pregnancy. Proper diet supports the baby's growth and development, while exercise helps preserve overall health and well-being.

During pregnancy, your partner's dietary needs vary. She requires more key nutrients, such as folic acid, iron, calcium, and protein. A balanced diet rich in fruits, vegetables, whole grains, and lean meats is vital. Encourage her to eat a variety of nutrient-dense foods and remain hydrated.

For example, folic acid is vital for preventing neural tube abnormalities in the infant. Encourage her to eat foods rich in folic acid, such as leafy greens, beans, and fortified cereals. Iron is vital for preventing anemia, so include iron-rich foods like lean meats, spinach, and legumes in her diet. Calcium promotes the baby's developing bones and teeth, so make sure she receives adequate dairy or fortified plant-based alternatives.

In addition to a healthy diet, taking prenatal vitamins as advised by her healthcare professional can assist ensure she obtains all the required nutrients. Be helpful by helping her remember to take these vitamins regularly.

Exercise is another key component of health and fitness throughout pregnancy. Regular physical activity can help alleviate pregnancy-related discomforts, boost mood, and increase general health. Encourage your spouse to engage in safe, moderate exercise, such as walking, swimming, or pregnant yoga. These activities can assist improve circulation, reduce edema, and alleviate back pain.

For instance, a daily stroll might be a terrific opportunity for both of you to be active and spend some quality time together. Prenatal yoga programs can also be useful, as they focus on moderate stretching and relaxation techniques adapted to the requirements of pregnant women.

It's crucial to contact her healthcare provider before starting any fitness program to ensure it's safe for her situation. Some activities may need to be changed or avoided, depending on her health and the stage of pregnancy.

Staying active can also have positive implications on emotional well-being. Exercise releases endorphins, which can help relieve stress and enhance happiness. Encouraging your partner to be active and join her in these activities can make the experience more joyful and supportive.

Hydration is another vital part of wellness throughout pregnancy. Proper hydration promotes the increased blood volume and amniotic fluid levels needed for a healthy pregnancy. Encourage her to drink plenty of water throughout the day. You can help by keeping a water bottle handy and reminding her to drink regularly.

Rest and sleep are also vital for physical and emotional well-being. As the pregnancy progresses, your partner may find it tough to get comfortable at night. Support her by establishing a sleep-friendly environment. This can involve utilizing extra pillows for support, keeping the bedroom cold and dark, and establishing a peaceful bedtime routine.

For example, you could assist her arrange pillows to support her back and belly or raise her legs to prevent edema. Encouraging a consistent sleep routine and reducing screen time before bed can help promote better sleep.

Supporting your partner's health and welfare throughout pregnancy involves a combination of understanding, empathy, and practical acts. By being informed about the changes her body is going through, providing emotional support, and encouraging healthy habits, you may play a significant role in ensuring a healthy and joyful pregnancy experience. Remember, the route to motherhood is a shared adventure, and your involvement makes a major difference. Together, you can traverse this changing moment with confidence and love. Welcome to the rewarding journey of supporting your partner and preparing for the arrival of your kid.

Chapter 4: Tests and Visits with Doctors (ANTENATAL)

Prenatal exams and doctor visits are essential components of a healthy pregnancy. They guarantee that both the mother's health and the baby's development are on the correct path by offering insightful information. You can assist your spouse and remain informed throughout the pregnancy journey as an expectant father if you know what to anticipate at these sessions and the importance of certain tests and screenings.

Prenatal visits are routine examinations with a medical professional to track the mother's and the unborn child's health as well as the pregnancy's progress. In the first and second trimesters, these visits usually take place once a month; as the due date draws near, they subsequently happen every two weeks, and finally once a week.

The medical professional will perform several standard examinations throughout these visits. They will take your partner's blood pressure and weight as one of their initial tasks. Since both too little and too much weight gain can endanger the pregnancy, it is crucial to keep an eye on weight gain to make sure it stays within a healthy range. Blood pressure is measured to keep an eye out for diseases like preeclampsia, which can be dangerous if left untreated.

Monitoring the baby's heartbeat is another standard procedure during prenatal visits. A portable Doppler gadget can be used for this. When you hear your baby's heartbeat for the first time, it's a wonderful feeling and a comforting indication that your pregnancy is going well.

The fundal height, or the distance between the pubic bone and the top of the uterus, will be measured by the healthcare professional as the pregnancy goes on. This measurement aids in monitoring the infant's development and growth. Additionally, particularly in the latter stages of pregnancy, they could feel the abdomen to ascertain the location of the baby.

Regular urine tests will also be performed on your partner during these sessions. These tests look for glucose levels, which can show gestational diabetes, protein levels, which can show preeclampsia, and infection symptoms. Additionally, routine blood tests are performed to determine the mother's blood type and Rh factor, as well as to check for diseases like anemia.

Your partner can also talk to the healthcare practitioner about any symptoms or worries during prenatal visits. Urge her to express any concerns or uneasiness she may be feeling. A healthy pregnancy can be ensured by taking proactive measures to alleviate issues.

During pregnancy, your spouse may have several common tests and screenings in addition to standard examinations. Important details regarding the health and development of the infant are revealed by these tests.

The blood test to determine hormone levels and confirm pregnancy is one of the initial tests. Usually, this test is performed at the first prenatal appointment. It helps create a care plan for the pregnancy and gives you baseline data on your partner's health.

Your spouse may have a nuchal translucency (NT) screening between weeks 10 and 14 of pregnancy. The thickness of the fluid at the back of the baby's neck is measured by this ultrasound examination. Increased thickness may indicate Down syndrome or other chromosomal disorders. To increase the accuracy of the results, a blood test is frequently included in the NT screening.

Non-invasive prenatal testing (NIPT) is another crucial screening method. By examining fetal DNA in the mother's blood, this blood test, which can be performed as early as the tenth week of pregnancy, checks for chromosomal abnormalities. In addition to being extremely accurate, NIPT can identify the baby's sex.

Your spouse may have the quadruple screen (quad screen) test between weeks 15 and 20 of pregnancy. This blood test evaluates the mother's blood for four distinct chemicals to determine her chance of developing birth defects, such as trisomy 18, neural tube disorders, and Down

syndrome. The quad screen can show whether additional testing is required, but it is not a diagnostic tool.

To screen for gestational diabetes, your partner will also have a glucose test as the pregnancy goes on. Typically, this test is conducted between weeks 24 and 28 of pregnancy. After an hour, your partner's blood sugar levels will be checked after she consumes a sugary solution. To identify gestational diabetes, additional testing could be required if the results are high.

Another crucial test is the group B streptococcus (GBS) screening, which is usually conducted between weeks 35 and 37 of pregnancy. GBS is a type of bacteria that can cause serious illnesses and be transferred to the infant after birth. In order to lower the danger of transmission to the unborn child, your partner will get antibiotics during labor if she tests positive for GBS.

Another crucial aspect of the prenatal care process is comprehending ultrasound and other imaging examinations. Using sound waves, ultrasound is a non-invasive imaging method that produces pictures of the unborn child. It is frequently used to track the growth and development of the unborn child during pregnancy.

Between weeks eight and fourteen of pregnancy is when the first ultrasound, also known as the dating ultrasound, is typically conducted.

This ultrasound aids in determining the due date, confirming the pregnancy, and determining whether more than one baby is present. When

you see the baby's tiny heartbeat for the first time, you feel so happy and reassured.

The anatomy scan, which usually takes place between weeks 18 and 22, is the next significant ultrasound. The baby's anatomy, including the brain, heart, spine, and other critical organs, is examined in this comprehensive scan. If you want to know, it can also tell the baby's sex. The anatomy scan can identify any possible anomalies and offers crucial information about the baby's growth.

Additional ultrasounds could occasionally be required to track the baby's development and position, particularly if there are worries regarding the baby's size or the quantity of amniotic fluid. The placenta's position and proper operation can also be checked with ultrasounds.

Magnetic resonance imaging (MRI) is another imaging modality that may be employed during pregnancy. MRI produces fine-grained images of the mother's and the baby's interior structures using radio waves and magnetic fields. It is usually employed when a problem that cannot be thoroughly evaluated by ultrasound requires more specific information for diagnosis or monitoring.

For instance, an MRI might be advised if the placenta is positioned in a way that could make delivery more difficult or if there are worries about the baby's brain development. Pregnancy-related MRIs are thought to be safe and offer useful information without exposing the mother or unborn child to radiation.

Being aware of these medical procedures, examinations, and imaging methods as an expectant father enables you to support your spouse and remain involved in the pregnancy process. Making every effort to attend her prenatal checkups demonstrates your dedication and gives you a chance to ask questions and find out more about the growth of the unborn child.

Medical examinations and tests are an integral component of prenatal care, offering vital information for both the mother's and the unborn child's health and growth. You will feel more prepared and confident as an expectant father if you know what to anticipate at these appointments, the importance of routine tests and screenings, and the function of ultrasound and other imaging modalities. Your participation and support are crucial to ensuring that you and your spouse have a happy and healthy pregnancy experience. Welcome to the thrilling path of motherhood, where you will eventually meet your child at every turn.

Chapter 5: The Experience of a Pregnant Partner

Many physical, emotional, and psychological changes occur during pregnancy, making it a life-changing period. It's essential to comprehend these changes and how they affect your partner to provide her with the understanding and support she requires. This chapter will explore the many experiences of a pregnant partner, emphasizing the physical, emotional, and psychological changes as well as useful strategies for being a sympathetic and encouraging partner.

The Physical Alterations and Their Impact on Your Spouse

The body undergoes a number of significant physical changes during pregnancy as it prepares to sustain the developing baby. Your partner may experience both positive and negative effects from these changes.

An increase in breast size and sensitivity is among the first physical changes your spouse may notice. Hormonal changes that prime the body for breastfeeding are the cause of this. She might notice that her areolas are swollen, sensitive, and even black. It's crucial to be kind and empathetic when she brings up this sensitivity, and wearing a supportive bra can assist ease discomfort.

The most obvious change as the pregnancy goes on is the expanding belly. The abdomen stretches and enlarges as the uterus grows to accommodate the growing baby. Itching and straining of the skin may result from this. Reducing irritation and soothing the skin can be achieved by using a moisturizing lotion or oil. Furthermore, the weight of the developing baby may place strain on the pelvis and back, resulting in posture abnormalities and back pain.

Gaining weight is a normal and essential aspect of pregnancy. In addition to providing energy reserves for birthing and breastfeeding, it promotes the baby's growth. But the extra weight might lead to exhaustion and physical strain. Weight gain can be controlled and general health can be enhanced by encouraging your partner to eat a balanced diet and do mild exercise.

Another typical physical alteration that occurs during pregnancy is swelling, which is also referred to as edema. Because of the increased volume of blood and fluid, it frequently affects the hands, ankles, and feet. Swelling can be lessened by elevating her feet, drinking plenty of water, and wearing cozy shoes. If she needs to change her activities or take additional breaks, be patient and empathetic.

Gastrointestinal problems including heartburn, nausea, vomiting (morning sickness), and constipation can also be brought on by hormonal changes.

Certain foods or scents might cause morning sickness, which usually happens in the first trimester. Avoiding strong scents and promoting small, frequent meals can help control nausea. Eating smaller meals, avoiding fatty or spicy foods, and drinking enough water might help relieve constipation and heartburn.

Due to the growing baby pressing against the diaphragm, your partner may have dyspnea as the pregnancy goes on. Simple tasks may feel more taxing as a result. To assist her breathing easier, encourage her to take breaks, stay away from physically demanding activities, and engage in deep breathing techniques.

Changes in Emotion and Psychology During Pregnancy

Pregnancy can cause a variety of emotional and psychological changes in addition to physical ones. An emotional rollercoaster can result from hormonal changes and the excitement of becoming a parent.

Mood swings are a typical emotional shift. Estrogen and progesterone are two important hormones that affect mood, and changes in these hormones during pregnancy can cause abrupt emotional shifts. Your partner might experience anxiety or tears one moment, followed by feelings of excitement and joy the next. It's critical to acknowledge that these mood fluctuations are a typical aspect of pregnancy and to exercise patience and compassion.

Stress and worry can also be brought on by pregnancy. Anxiety can be increased by the prospect of parenthood, worries about the health of the unborn child, and physical changes in your partner. Some of these concerns can be avoided by promoting candid communication and offering confidence. For instance, going to childbirth classes with her and talking about the birth plan can help her feel more in control and prepared if she's nervous about the delivery.

The nesting instinct is another typical emotional response during pregnancy. Your partner could have a great desire to get the house ready for the baby's birth as the due date draws near. This can involve making sure everything is in its proper place, cleaning, and organizing the nursery. By assisting her with these preparations, you may support her nesting instincts and foster a happy atmosphere.

Changes in body image and self-consciousness are other effects of pregnancy. Your girlfriend can become less self-assured about her appearance as her body changes. Positive affirmations and reassurance that she is lovely and that these changes are normal during pregnancy are crucial. Telling her how much you value her and the amazing work her body is doing, for example, might help her feel more confident and good about herself.

How to Be a Compassionate and Helpful Partner

Understanding the changes your spouse is going through and providing both practical and emotional support are key components of being an understanding and encouraging partner during pregnancy.

Active listening is one of the best strategies to help your relationship. When she shares her feelings, worries, or experiences, listens carefully without interjecting or providing answers right away. Sometimes all she needs is someone to listen to her and validate her feelings. For instance, validate her sentiments and reassure her that it's acceptable if she expresses anger about her changing physique.

Another important component of assistance is offering physical comfort. Provide back massages to ease back pain, use cushions to help her find comfortable resting positions, and aid her with bending and lifting duties. Little things like setting up a comfortable place for her to unwind or running a warm bath can have a significant impact on her comfort.

Promoting healthful behaviors is also crucial. Together, prepare wholesome meals to help her maintain a balanced diet. Participate in mild activities with her, like walking or prenatal yoga, to help her feel better physically and emotionally. In addition to improving her health, staying active together gives them a chance to spend time together and form bonds.

Stress reduction is essential for her mental health. Assist her in discovering methods to decompress, including going for a stroll in the outdoors, spending a peaceful evening at home, or engaging in mindfulness and meditation. Provide a serene, encouraging atmosphere while keeping in mind her emotional requirements.

Attending prenatal classes and appointments demonstrates your interest and dedication to the pregnancy process. Ask inquiries, keep up with the baby's progress, and accompany her to doctor's appointments whenever you can. Prenatal programs offer useful knowledge and skills that will make you both feel more equipped to give birth and raise a family.

It's important to show your affection and gratitude. Knowing that you value her sacrifices and efforts can help her feel better throughout the difficult time that is pregnancy. Your relationship can be strengthened and she will feel appreciated by small actions like telling her how much you love her, hugging her, or writing a loving note.

Lastly, exercise flexibility and adaptability. Unexpected events abound throughout pregnancy, so it's critical to be flexible and supportive when required. Being sympathetic and patient will help a lot, whether it's a last-minute craving, an emotional outburst, or an unforeseen day of rest.

A variety of physical, emotional, and psychological changes occur during the pregnant partner's experience. Being aware of these changes and how they affect your partner enables you to provide her with the understanding and support she requires. You may foster a healthy and supportive atmosphere for your partner and your developing child by actively listening, providing emotional and physical support, promoting healthy habits, and showing your love and gratitude. Together, you can face this life-changing experience with courage, love, and fortitude. Welcome to the amazing path of parenting, where you are getting closer to the birth of your child every second.

Chapter 6: Delivery Preparation

One of the most exciting and important aspects of pregnancy is getting ready for the birth of your child. It's critical to have a well-defined plan and be ready for the big day as the deadline draws near. Creating a birth plan, getting ready for the hospital or birthing facility, and packing the necessities for the hospital bag are all covered in this chapter. You and your spouse can have a more seamless and satisfying delivery experience if you are well-prepared and organized.

A birth plan is a written statement of your choices and preferences for the course of labor and delivery. It ensures that everyone is aware of your desires by acting as a communication tool between you, your spouse, and the medical staff. Although flexibility is crucial, having a birth plan can help people feel more in control and less anxious.

Think about a number of choices and possibilities that will affect your experience when making a birth plan. Where you want to give birth is one of your first decisions. Talk to your spouse about whether you would rather give birth at home, in a hospital, or in a birthing center. Every choice offers a unique set of advantages and things to think about. For example, birthing facilities offer a more homelike setting with fewer medical interventions, yet hospitals offer prompt medical assistance in the event of difficulties.

Next, consider how you would like to manage your pain. There are some treatments, including medical interventions like epidurals and analgesics as well as natural pain management therapies like massage, hydrotherapy, and breathing exercises. To find the option that best suits your requirements and tastes, talk about these alternatives with your partner and healthcare provider.

Having support persons around is another crucial component of your birth plan. Choose your partner to accompany you through labor and delivery. This might be a doula, your spouse, a friend, or a member of your family. A skilled expert who offers both physical and emotional support during childbirth is known as a doula. Being with someone who is encouraging can have a big impact on your confidence and comfort level.

Think about your choices for mobility and work positions. Walking, squatting, or using a birthing ball are some of the ways that some women choose to move during labor. Others might be more at ease in a semi-reclined position or lying down. Talk to your healthcare practitioner about these possibilities and see which one suits you the best.

Additionally, consider your preferences for procedures like intravenous fluids, continuous fetal monitoring, and, if necessary, the use of forceps or vacuum extraction. You should be receptive to medical advice, but you may also make better decisions if you know exactly what you want.

Following discussion and decision-making on these points, clearly and succinctly draft your birth plan. To make sure that everyone knows your desires, share them with your healthcare physician and the staff at the hospital or birthing center. Keep in mind that flexibility is essential and that the birth plan is not final. Being flexible will enable you to handle unforeseen circumstances with assurance.

To guarantee a seamless and well-organized experience, there are several practical things to do before arriving at the hospital or birthing facility. Touring the facilities is one of the first things to do. This will acquaint you with the layout, the facilities that are offered, and the rules and regulations. Arriving at the hospital or birthing center might be more comfortable and anxiety-reducing if you know where to go and what to anticipate.

Pre-registering at the hospital or birthing facility is also crucial. This entails completing the required forms and supplying your insurance details beforehand. When you come for delivery, pre-registering might help you save time and feel less stressed. A few weeks before the deadline, finish this stage and inquire with the facility about any special requirements.

Talking about travel plans is still another important component. When labor starts, make plans for how you will go to the hospital or birthing facility. Take into account the distance from your house, the time of day, and the traffic. Having a backup plan in place is also a smart idea. For example, you may have a friend or family member drive you in an emergency.

One of the most important aspects of getting ready for birth is packing the hospital bag. It might be more relaxed and pleasant if you have everything you need on hand. To avoid rushing at the last minute, begin packing the hospital bag a few weeks before the due date. This is a comprehensive list of what needs to be included:

Regarding the Partner in Childbirth

Comfortable attire: Bring loose, relaxed clothing for the hospital stay, labor, and delivery. Think about packing a pair of comfortable socks, slippers, and a robe.

Toiletries such as toothpaste and toothbrush, shampoo, conditioner, soap, hairbrush, deodorant, and any other personal care products you use on a regular basis should be included. During labor, lips can become dry, so remember to apply lip balm.

Crucial documents: Your ID, insurance card, and other required documents, such as your birth plan and hospital pre-registration forms, should be brought.

beverages and snacks: Having beverages and snacks on hand will help you stay energized during the lengthy workday. Bring water or sports drinks, as well as light snacks like granola bars, nuts, and dried fruit. Although some hospitals offer meals, it's beneficial to have your own choices.

- **Entertainment**: Bring a book, magazine, iPad, or music player with headphones to help you kill time. In the early stages of labor, these might be a pleasant diversion.

Phone and charger: To stay in contact with loved ones and to record those initial priceless moments with your child, remember to bring along your phone and a charger.

For the infant:

Clothes: Bring a couple of clothing for the infant, including one for when they return home. Select clothing that is simple to put on and take off, including sleepers and onesies. Remember to provide the infant with hats, mittens, and socks to keep them warm.

Blankets: Pack a few nice, soft blankets to swaddle and keep the infant warm.

Diapers and wipes: Although the hospital typically supplies these items, it's a good idea to pack some of your own in case you need them.

Car seat: Before the deadline, confirm that the car seat is correctly placed in your vehicle. Make sure you understand how to use the car seat properly by bringing the manual.

For the Supporting Person (Breasting Partner):

comfy attire: Bring personal belongings and comfy clothing for your hospital stay. Because hospital temperatures might vary, wear layers.

Drinks and snacks: Pack enough water and food to keep you alert and energized. It can be difficult to be a supportive birthing partner, so having food on hand will make things easier.

 Entertainment: Bring along a book, iPad, or music player to keep you busy during the slower times.

Phone and charger: To stay in touch with loved ones, make sure you have your phone and a charger.

Make sure the hospital bag is in a convenient location as the due date draws near. Store it in a handy place, like the car or by the door, so you can get to it fast when labor starts.

Careful planning and doable actions are necessary to create a seamless and satisfying delivery experience. Important components of this preparation include making a birth plan, getting ready for the hospital or birthing facility, and packing the hospital bag. You can provide your partner the consolation and support they require during this important time if you are well-prepared and structured. Together, you may face the birthing process with enthusiasm and confidence, knowing that you are ready for your baby's arrival. Welcome to the amazing journey of motherhood, where you get closer to meeting your child every second.

Chapter 7: Delivery and Labor

The culmination of the pregnancy journey, which is characterized by joy, anticipation, and sometimes some anxiety, is labor and delivery. You may support your spouse during this important time by being aware of the stages of labor, the indications of labor, and your role in the delivery room. This chapter will walk you through each of these areas, making sure you feel ready and secure as your baby's birth draws near.

When to Visit the Hospital for Labor Signs

The first step in determining when to go to the hospital or birthing facility is recognizing the signs of labor. Some physical symptoms that signal your partner's body is preparing for childbirth usually precede labor. Here are some important indicators to look out for:

Regular contractions are one of the most typical indicators of labor. True labor contractions are regular, intensify, and happen at regular intervals, in contrast to Braxton Hicks contractions, which are erratic and frequently painless. Usually, they begin in the lower back and progress to the abdomen's front. Time them from the beginning of one contraction to the beginning of the next to see whether they are the real thing. It's necessary to contact the healthcare provider and go to the hospital if they are occurring every five minutes and lasting for at least an hour.

Water Breaking: The rupture of the amniotic sac, which releases the fluid enveloping the baby, is another obvious indication of labor. This may occur as a gradual trickle or as an abrupt burst of fluid. If your partner's water breaks, make a note of the fluid's color and smell; the medical professional will need to know this information. Even if contractions have not yet begun, it is imperative to visit the hospital as soon as the water breaks since once the sac is ruptured, there is a greater chance of infection.

Bloody Show: The "bloody show" is a pink or bloody discharge that your partner may detect in the later stages of pregnancy. This happens when the cervix's mucus plug is released, indicating that labor might start shortly. It's a sign that things are moving forward, but it doesn't necessarily indicate that labor is about to begin.

Lower Back Pain and Pelvic Pressure: Your partner may feel lower back pain and pelvic pressure as the baby is ready to be born. This pain is frequently an indication that labor is about to begin. It's wise to get in touch with the healthcare practitioner if the pain is severe and accompanied by further labor symptoms.

Nesting Instinct: In the days preceding labor, some women feel a surge of energy and a need to tidy and arrange their houses. This "nesting instinct" may be a sign that the body is getting ready for the big event, but it is not a clear indication of labor.

It might be difficult to know when to visit the hospital, particularly if it's your first time. If you're unsure, it's always best to be careful and get in

touch with the healthcare practitioner. They can assist you choose whether it's time to visit the hospital and offer advice based on the symptoms.

The Labor Stages and What to Anticipate

There are three primary phases of labor: the first, which includes transition, active labor, and early labor; the second, which involves pushing and delivery; and the third, which involves placenta delivery. You can encourage your partner and maintain your composure by being aware of what to anticipate at each stage.

First Phase: Transition, Active Labor, and Early Labor.

Early Labor: Especially for first-time mothers, early labor, which marks the start of the first stage, can linger for several hours or even days. The cervix starts to dilate and efface (thin out) in the early stages of labor. Usually lasting 30 to 45 seconds and happening every 5 to 30 minutes, contractions are mild to moderate and erratic. Your significant other might experience anxiety, excitement, or both. To maintain her energy levels, encourage her to take breaks, drink plenty of water, and eat small snacks. Discomfort can be managed by walking, having a warm shower, or using relaxation methods.

Active Labor: The more intense stage that follows the first is called active labor. Contractions are stronger, more frequent, and closer together as the cervix dilates by 6 to 10 cm. They last for roughly 60 seconds and happen every 3 to 5 minutes. If you haven't been to the hospital yet, now is the moment. The medical staff at the hospital will keep an eye on your companion and assess her condition. Whether it's holding her hand, giving

her ice chips, or assisting her in finding comfortable positions, provide constant support throughout active labor. Massages and breathing techniques can also aid with pain management.

Transition: The last and most intense part of the first stage is transition. Strong contractions that last 60 to 90 seconds and happen every two to three minutes occur as the cervix dilates by 8 to 10 cm. During this time, your partner might feel overburdened, agitated, or worn out. Assure her that the most difficult phase is almost over and that she is doing a fantastic job. Maintaining composure and offering support can assist her in overcoming this difficult phase.

Stage Two: Pushing and Delivering

until the cervix is 10 centimeters dilated, the second stage of labor starts, and it concludes until the baby is born. Depending on many variables, this period may last a few minutes to several hours.

Every contraction in the second stage will make your spouse want to push. She will receive advice from the healthcare professional on when and how to push successfully. It's important to find the ideal pushing position. Some women would rather lie on their side, squat, or use a birthing stool. Urge your significant other to pay attention to her body and heed the advice of the medical staff.

The medical professional will keep an eye on the mother's and the baby's health while they pass through the delivery canal. You can be requested to offer words of encouragement, water, or assistance for your partner's legs.

There is a great deal of excitement when the baby crowns, or when its head is revealed. Tell your partner that the baby is on the verge of arriving.

The infant will be placed on your partner's chest for instant skin-to-skin contact by the healthcare professional once the baby is born. This aids in controlling the infant's breathing, heart rate, and temperature. Additionally, it's a lovely time for the parents to bond. After clamping and cutting the umbilical cord, the medical professional will make sure the mother and child are stable and healthy.

Stage Three: Placenta Delivery

The placenta is delivered during the third stage of labor. Usually, this happens five to thirty minutes after the baby is born. As the uterus contracts to release the placenta, your partner may feel minor contractions during this period. The medical professional will make sure there are no issues and that the placenta is delivered whole.

The medical staff will keep an eye out for any indications of severe bleeding or other issues once the placenta is delivered. If necessary, they will also clean and sew any rips or episiotomies. Encourage your partner to take it easy and savor the early days spent with your child.

How You Function in the Delivery Room

In the delivery room, your job as a birthing partner is to help the woman emotionally, physically, and practically. Your partner's experience can be greatly improved by being a soothing and composed presence. You can help her during labor and delivery in the following ways:

Emotional Support: Constantly reassure and encourage. Tell your spouse that you are supporting her at every turn and that she is doing a fantastic job. "You're doing great," "I'm so proud of you," and "Our baby will be here soon" are examples of simple affirmations that can give you more strength and confidence.

Physical Support: Assist your spouse in locating postures that will be pleasant during labor and delivery. This could be reclining on her side, walking, or utilizing a birthing ball. Hold her hand while she contracts, give her a massage, or counter-press her lower back. Be patient and offer gentle assistance if she wishes to shift positions or move about.

Be ready to offer practical support, such as obtaining a warm compress, changing the pillows, or grabbing ice chips. Offer her water or other clear liquids to stay hydrated. Whether she needs essential oils, a familiar object from home, or her favorite song, make sure she has access to it.

Advocacy: Speak up in favor of your partner's birth plan and preferences. If necessary, speak with the medical staff on her behalf and make sure her desires are honored. Ask questions and go over the alternatives with your partner and the healthcare provider if any medical measures are recommended.

Seizing the Moment: Take pictures or videos of the memorable moments if your partner requests it. We will treasure these memories for years to come. Nonetheless, always honors her desires and the hospital's recording and photographic guidelines.

Remaining composed: The process of giving birth can be stressful and uncertain. If things don't go as planned, maintain your composure. Your composed manner might reduce your partner's nervousness and foster a happier environment.

Post-Delivery Support: Continue to offer assistance during the recuperation phase following the baby's birth. Help with baby care duties like changing diapers and swaddling, as well as breastfeeding if she decides to do so. Urge your significant other to rest and look after herself.

Labor and delivery are important turning points in the pregnancy process. You may give your spouse tremendous assistance if you know the stages of labor, the indications of labor, and your role in the delivery room. Both of you will have a great and empowered birth experience because of your presence, support, and helpful advice. Together, you may joyfully, confidently, and lovingly welcome your baby into the world. Best wishes on

Chapter 8: The Time After Giving Birth

The fourth trimester, sometimes referred to as the postpartum phase, is a time of major transition and adjustment for both the mother and the infant. Recuperation, bonding, and adjusting to the new dynamics of motherhood are all part of this time. Supporting breastfeeding and infant feeding decisions, knowing the mental landscape, including postpartum depression and anxiety, and knowing what to anticipate throughout postpartum recovery can all help you give your spouse the best care possible.

Recognizing Your Partner's Postpartum Recuperation

The physical strain of pregnancy and delivery will cause your partner's body to undergo a healing process after giving birth. Although each woman's recovery time is unique, many go through similar experiences and changes.

Your partner may have lochia, or postpartum hemorrhage, in the initial days following delivery. This can continue for a few weeks and is the body's method of removing the uterine lining. Like a heavy menstrual period, the bleeding will begin heavy and bright red and then progressively lighten in color and flow. Make sure your significant other has lots of maternity pads and cozy underwear. Tampon use should be avoided during this period to lower the risk of infection.

After giving birth, pain and discomfort are typical, particularly if your partner delivered the baby vaginally. Tearing or an episiotomy may cause her to feel sore in the perineal region, which is the space between the vagina and anus. Pain can be reduced by using ice packs, having sitz baths, and taking over-the-counter painkillers. She will require particular care for the site of her incision if she has a cesarean section. It is crucial to keep the area dry and clean and to adhere to the wound care guidelines given by the healthcare professional.

As your partner gets ready to breastfeed, their breasts will also undergo modifications. Her breasts may feel swollen and sore in the initial days after delivery as they swell with milk. Although it may cause discomfort, this is a typical step in the process. To ease engorgement, encourage her to use a breast pump or to breastfeed more regularly. Pain can be lessened by applying cold compresses after nursing and warm compresses before.

Postpartum healing is significantly influenced by hormonal changes. Mood swings, exhaustion, and changes in energy levels might result from the quick decline in pregnancy hormones following delivery. The "baby blues," which include depressive, irritable, and emotionally sensitive moods, are prevalent among new mothers. After birth, these emotions typically reach their zenith a few days later and then go away in two weeks. It's critical to offer compassion and emotional support during this time.

Sleep and rest are essential for healing, but they can be difficult to provide for a newborn. Because of their erratic sleep schedules and frequent feedings, newborns can wear out your companion. Encourage her to nap when the baby is napping and to rest whenever she can. She can receive much-needed sleep by sharing nocturnal tasks like changing the baby's diaper and calming her.

Another important factor in postpartum healing is nutrition. To encourage breastfeeding and promote healing, your partner's body requires additional nutrients. Urge her to have a well-rounded diet full of lean proteins, healthy grains, fruits, and vegetables. It's equally crucial to stay hydrated, particularly if she's nursing. You can make sure she's getting the nutrients she needs by offering to cook for her or by bringing her wholesome snacks and beverages.

Encouragement of Breastfeeding and Choices for Infant Feeding

Although breastfeeding is a healthy and natural way to feed a baby, there are some drawbacks. Your assistance can have a big impact on your partner's breastfeeding experience.

Learning about the procedure and advantages of breastfeeding is one of the first steps towards promoting it. Antibodies and vital nutrients included in breast milk help shield the infant from diseases and infections.

Additionally, it strengthens the mother-child relationship. Knowing the fundamentals of breastfeeding, including latching methods, feeding positions, and typical problems, can enable you to offer helpful assistance. It's critical to support and encourage your spouse to use appropriate breastfeeding techniques. For breastfeeding to be successful and to avoid nipple pain and injury, a good latch is necessary. Make sure the infant and your spouse are both in a comfortable posture and that the areola—the black region surrounding the nipple—is mostly covered by the baby's mouth. Consider getting assistance from a lactation consultant if she is having pain or trouble latching; they can offer knowledgeable advice and support.

Establishing a healthy milk supply in the early stages requires frequent feeding. When the baby exhibits symptoms of hunger, such as rooting, sucking on hands, or fussiness, encourage your partner to nurse on demand. It can be draining for newborns to feed every two to three hours. You can allow your partner time to rest and recuperate by offering to help with other chores or to watch the baby in between feedings.

Establishing a breastfeeding-friendly workplace is also crucial. Make sure your spouse has a cozy space with water, snacks, and pillows for nursing. She can concentrate better on nursing and developing a bond with the baby if she is less stressed and distracted.

Your assistance is just as crucial if your spouse decides to pump breast milk. Assist her with feeding the infant, storing extracted milk appropriately, and setting up and cleaning the breast pump. Breast milk can be kept safe and nourishing for the infant by following the proper handling and storage instructions.

Despite the many advantages of breastfeeding, it's crucial to recognize and encourage your partner's feeding preferences, whether they involve formula, breastfeeding, or a mix of the two. Some mothers may opt to use formula for personal reasons or encounter obstacles that make breastfeeding challenging. The baby's health and nutrition are the most important factors.

Learn about the many kinds of formula and how to properly prepare and store it if your partner chooses to formula feed. To allow your partner to relax and recuperate, offer to assist with bottle feedings. Keep in mind that feeding is also a chance for bonding, and bottle feeding allows you to develop deep relationships with your infant.

The Emotional Environment: Anxiety and Postpartum Depression

Many new mothers experience a range of feelings throughout the postpartum period, which can be an emotional rollercoaster. The "baby blues," which are transient mood fluctuations and feelings of sadness, are typical, but some moms may endure more serious illnesses like anxiety and postpartum depression.

Approximately one in seven new mothers suffer from postpartum depression (PPD), a dangerous illness. It is characterized by enduring feelings of melancholy, pessimism, and a lack of interest in once-enjoyable activities and can happen at any point within the first year following childbirth. Changes in appetite and sleep patterns, trouble bonding with the baby, and suicidal thoughts are some other signs. Recognizing the symptoms and encouraging your spouse to get expert care are key components of supporting her through postpartum depression.

Discussing these issues with her is crucial if you observe that she is exhibiting signs of post-traumatic stress disorder (PPD), such as ongoing unhappiness, social disengagement, or trouble adjusting to daily life. Urge her to speak with her doctor, who can offer a correct diagnosis and suggest therapies like counseling, medicine, or support groups.

Another ailment that can impact new mothers is postpartum anxiety. In addition to feeling overburdened by the responsibilities of motherhood, it entails excessive worry, fear, and anxiety over the health and safety of the unborn child. Constant concern, restlessness, physical symptoms like lightheadedness or a fast heartbeat, and trouble falling asleep are all common signs of postpartum anxiety.

Providing comfort and useful assistance is essential to helping your partner cope with postpartum anxiety. Validate her sentiments and encourage her to discuss her worries and fears. Her stress levels can be lowered by assisting with baby care duties and fostering a serene, encouraging environment. Encourage her to get professional assistance if her anxiety becomes too much to handle.

It's critical to keep in mind that anxiety and postpartum depression are medical disorders that call for care and assistance. Your comprehension and support can have a big impact on your partner's healing.

You can support your partner's emotional health in addition to seeking expert assistance by taking the following doable actions:

Promote Self-Care: Mental wellness depends on self-care. Whether it's a peaceful moment with a book, a walk, or a warm bath, encourage your partner to take some time for herself. She can feel more capable and balanced if she takes care of her own needs.

Provide Assistance and Support: Take the initiative to provide assistance with household chores and baby care. Little acts of kindness like preparing a meal, doing the laundry, or watching the infant so she can sleep can have a significant impact.

Keep in Touch: Motivate your significant other to maintain relationships with friends and family. Emotional health depends on social support. Make plans to see or speak with loved ones who can offer support and company.

Encourage your significant other to uphold healthy routines, such as eating wholesome meals, drinking enough water, and exercising frequently. Mental and physical health are intimately related.

Be understanding and patient: It takes time to recover from postpartum anxiety and sadness. Show your girlfriend that you are there for her at every turn by being understanding and patient with her. Don't assign blame or pass judgment; instead, show compassion and empathy.

Major emotional and physical changes occur during the postpartum phase. To provide your spouse with the most support possible, you must understand postpartum healing, encourage breastfeeding and infant feeding choices, and recognize the symptoms of postpartum depression and anxiety. You can contribute to creating a supportive and caring atmosphere for your partner and your child by being proactive, knowledgeable, and sympathetic. By working together, you may successfully negotiate the pleasures and difficulties of the postpartum phase and create a solid basis for your new family.

Chapter 9: The Initial Weeks Of New Baby

Your newborn's first few weeks are a time of amazing change, adjustment, and happiness. Even though it can be overwhelming at times, you and your infant can have a more seamless transition if you know what to anticipate and develop routines. New fathers also need to put self-care first to remain active and healthy. This chapter will help you navigate these initial weeks by offering helpful tips and insights.

First Days of a Baby: What to Expect

You experience a mixture of surprise, joy, and some degree of uncertainty in the initial days following bringing your newborn home. You can feel more prepared and confident if you know what to anticipate.

Newborns sleep for 16 to 18 hours a day, which is one of the first things you'll notice. Nevertheless, this sleep is typically interrupted by brief intervals of two to four hours, resulting in numerous awakenings both during the day and at night. Resting whenever you can is crucial during this time because it's common to feel worn out and sleep-deprived. Another important task in these early days is feeding. Due to their small tummies, newborns must eat every two to three hours. It's crucial to make sure your infant is eating frequently and gaining weight, regardless of whether you decide to bottle-feed or breastfeed them. Breastfeeding can be difficult at first for both the mother and the infant. Be patient and encouraging, and if necessary, seek assistance from medical professionals or lactation consultants.

You'll also be busy taking care of your baby's diaper needs. You should anticipate changing your diapers eight to twelve times a day. To make sure your baby is getting enough food and water, keep an eye on the quantity of wet and dirty diapers. This can also assist you in identifying possible problems early on.

During the first few days, you also need to take care of your baby's umbilical cord stump. Until it falls off, which normally happens in a week or two, keep the area dry and clean. Get in touch with your healthcare practitioner if you observe any redness, swelling, or discharge.
You will begin to observe your newborn's distinct personality and cues while you tend to them. Observe their cues for pain, hunger, and tiredness. You will be better able to meet your baby's requirements if you can read these indications.

During these early days, bonding with your kid is crucial. Talk, hold, and cuddle with your infant for a while. In addition to fostering bonding, skin-to-skin contact can assist control your baby's body temperature and heart rate. To enjoy these unique moments and build a close emotional bond with your child, take turns with your partner.

Creating Schedules and Routines

Establishing routines can help your days feel more organized and predictable, even though the first few weeks could feel chaotic. In addition to making everyday chores easier for you, routines give your infant a sense of security.

A feeding schedule is among the first routines to be established. Aim for consistent feeding times whether you're bottle-feeding or nursing. Although newborns normally need to eat every two to three hours, they will eventually be able to go longer between feedings as they get older. To make sure your baby is receiving adequate nutrition, keep track of the times and lengths of your feedings.

Sleep schedules are also crucial. Newborns sleep a lot, although their sleep habits might vary. Establish a soothing bedtime ritual to assist your infant in understanding when it's time to go to sleep. This could be reading a calming story, taking a warm bath, or gently rocking. Make an effort to create a regular sleeping environment by maintaining a quiet, dark, and comfortable temperature.

Routines can also be beneficial when it comes to changing diapers. Change your baby's diaper frequently, particularly when they wake up from naps and after feedings. Diaper changes can be made more efficient by keeping a well-stocked diaper station with all the necessities, including diapers, wipes, creams, and a change of clothes.
You can also incorporate bathing your infant into your daily routine. A newborn normally only needs to be bathed two or three times a week.

Keep the bathwater warm but not hot, and use a mild, baby-safe soap. For both you and your infant, make bath time calming and pleasurable.
Routines are vital, but it's as critical to maintaining flexibility. Given how erratic newborns can be, your baby's needs may occasionally diverge from the norm. You will be able to handle these situations more easily if you are flexible and attentive to your baby's cues.

Self-Care's Significance for New Fathers

Because caring for a newborn is so demanding, it's simple for new fathers to put their own needs last. Nonetheless, putting self-care first is crucial for your health, your capacity to assist your relationship, and your ability to care for your child.

Getting enough sleep is one of the most important parts of self-care. New parents frequently experience sleep loss, but it's critical to figure out how to relax and rejuvenate. To make sure you both get some sleep, take naps when your infant is resting and divide up the chores at night with your spouse. Resting for even brief periods can have a big impact.

It's also critical to keep up a nutritious diet. When you're busy, it's easy to reach for unhealthy, fast snacks, but wholesome meals will provide you with the energy you need. A balanced diet rich in whole grains, lean meats, fruits, and veggies is what you should strive for. Drink lots of water all day long since staying hydrated is equally vital.
You may maintain your physical and emotional well-being by engaging in regular physical activity. Look for opportunities to move throughout the day, even if you don't have time for a full workout. Do some gentle

stretching, going for a stroll with your infant, or working out quickly at home. Exercise can improve your general well-being, lower stress levels, and elevate your mood.

Another essential component of self-care is emotional support. It's common to experience a range of emotions throughout the stressful adjustment to parenthood. Discuss your feelings and experiences with your spouse, and don't be afraid to ask friends, family, or a professional counselor for help if necessary. Participating in online communities or parenting groups can also offer beneficial connections and support.

It's crucial to take pauses and make time for oneself. Making time for things you enjoy is crucial, even when your baby's needs come first. Make time for self-care activities that help you feel refreshed, whether that means reading a book, watching a favorite show, or doing a hobby. Another crucial aspect of self-care is maintaining a relationship with your partner. Although becoming a parent can strengthen your bond, it can also cause stress and pressure. Even if it's only a few minutes of quality time every day, make time for one another. Together, celebrate the little wins, encourage one another, and share your experiences.

Understand that the initial weeks spent with your infant are a period of bonding, learning, and adjustment. This shift can be made easier and more pleasurable by being prepared, creating routines, and placing a higher priority on self-care. You can provide a loving and supportive environment for your expanding family by looking after yourself and attending to your infant's needs.

Chapter 10: Bonding with Your Infant As A Father

One of the most fulfilling aspects of fatherhood is developing a relationship with your newborn. Finding your special role as a new father, the value of skin-to-skin contact, and many ways to bond with your infant are all covered in this chapter. You can build a solid, long-lasting relationship with your child by comprehending and appreciating these factors.

How to Communicate with Your Infant

Making a connection with your newborn entails emotional and physical exchanges that promote safety and affection. Here are a few doable strategies to strengthen that connection:

Holding and cuddling: One of the most effective methods to establish a connection with your newborn is through physical touch. Your infant feels reassured and comforted when you hold and cuddle them. You can establish a feeling of intimacy by rocking your baby, holding them gently in your arms, or just having them lie on your chest. Your baby may find comfort in the warmth and cadence of your heartbeat, which will strengthen your bond.

Singing and Talking: Your voice is very soothing, even if your kid doesn't yet grasp what you're saying. Throughout the day, speak to your infant by explaining your activities, sharing anecdotes, or just conversing. It might also be calming to sing your favorite tunes or lullabies. Your voice enhances your emotional bond and aids in your baby's recognition.

Eye Contact: One of the most effective ways to express love and care for your infant is to make eye contact. While singing or conversing, hold your infant close and gaze into their eyes. Your infant gains a sense of comfort and trust from this nonverbal connection, which makes them feel acknowledged and appreciated.

Feeding Time: Whether you are bottle-feeding or your partner is nursing, feeding time is a great chance to strengthen your relationship. Talk quietly, keep your eyes on your infant, and hold them near. You can strengthen your relationship by feeding and comforting each other during this private time.

Bathing and changing diapers are two common caregiver duties that provide great chances for bonding. Take a positive approach to these duties and utilize them as opportunities to build relationships. Make eye contact, talk to your infant gently, and give them comforting touches.

Your infant will feel cherished and cared for as a result of these interactions.

Play and Exploration: Take part in easy play activities with your baby, such as displaying them colorful toys, belly time, or light tickling. Create an interesting and safe atmosphere to promote curiosity and inquiry. In addition to being enjoyable, playtime is crucial for both your bonding experience and your baby's growth.

Reading Together: Reading to your infant fosters early language development and is a great way to strengthen your relationship. Select novels with straightforward, rhythmic writing and vibrant illustrations. As you read and point to the pictures, keep your infant near. Both the visual stimulus and the sound of your voice can captivate your infant and deepen your bond.

The Value of Skin-to-Skin Interaction

Kangaroo care, or skin-to-skin contact, is putting your nude infant on your bare chest while you cover them with a blanket. This technique is a great approach to strengthen the link between the parents and the child and has many advantages for both parties.

Physical Benefits for the Baby: Touching your baby's skin helps control their respiration, heart rate, and body temperature. Your skin's warmth creates a stable environment, which is crucial for premature infants. Additionally, this interaction encourages the release of oxytocin, a hormone that fosters bonding and lowers stress.

Emotional Advantages for the Infant: Your infant will feel more protected and secure if they have skin-to-skin contact. Comfort comes

from the warmth of your body, the sound of your heartbeat, and the familiarity of your perfume. Better sleep and less weeping can result from this intimate interaction.

Benefits for Parents: The infant and the parents both benefit from skin-to-skin contact. It increases the release of oxytocin, which promotes bonding and love. Both you and your partner can benefit from this practice by feeling less stressed and more content.

Finding a comfortable position that allows you to recline a little is the first step in practicing skin-to-skin contact. To maintain a free airway, place your infant on your bare chest with their head turned to the side. To keep your infant warm, cover them with a blanket. You should stay in this position for at least half an hour so that you can both unwind and bond.

Identifying Your New Dad Role

Discovering your special role as a new father entails recognizing your advantages, accepting your obligations, and developing deep relationships with your child. Here are a few strategies for identifying and accepting your role:

Becoming an Active Caregiver: Developing your role and fostering a bond with your infant depends on your active involvement in their care. Assist with feeding, changing diapers, bathing, and calming your infant. By participating in these routine activities, you establish a solid, trustworthy bond with your child and become an essential part of their lives.

Developing a pattern: Creating a daily pattern gives you and your child structure and makes them feel safe. Establish regular feeding, sleeping, and playing schedules. This predictability creates a sense of stability and helps your infant know what to expect. To strengthen your presence and connection, engage in these routines, whether they be morning cuddles or the bedtime ritual.

Supporting Your Partner: One of your responsibilities as a new father is to assist your partner. Your baby will live in a balanced and peaceful environment if you work as a team. Assign tasks together and offer your partner emotional support. Your infant will feel safe and cared for by both parents if you present a united front.

Learning and Adapting: Being a parent is an ongoing learning experience. Be willing to pick up new abilities and adjust to your baby's evolving requirements. Read books, take parenting classes, and ask seasoned parents for assistance. Accept the learning curve and don't be scared of making errors. Your capacity to develop and adapt strengthens your position as a capable and devoted father.

Creating important Moments: Look for methods to spend time with your child that are important to you both. This may be a weekend excursion, a nightly storytime, or a morning stroll. These customs and practices deepen your relationship and create priceless memories. Your infant will learn to connect your love and presence with these memorable moments.

Emotional Bond: Developing a relationship involves more than just face-to-face communication. Observe your infant's indications and react to them with compassion and affection. Recognize and react to your baby's cues, such as smiles, coos, or cries. Your emotional presence creates a strong bond with your infant by making them feel heard and appreciated.

Being Present: Being alert and present is a priceless gift you can give your child in the hectic environment of today. During your time with your infant, put electronics and work aside as distractions. Give your youngster your whole attention and concentrate on the here and now. Giving your child your full attention improves your relationship and gives them a sense of security.

Sharing Your Interests: Share your hobbies and pastimes with your child. Sharing your interests, whether they be literature, sports, music, or the outdoors, fosters relationships. For instance, if you enjoy music, play an instrument and sing for your child. Take your infant on nature walks if you're an outdoor enthusiast. These common experiences strengthen your friendship and lay the groundwork for more bonding exercises in the future.

Active caregiving, emotional connection, and physical touch are all important components of developing a bond with your newborn. You build a solid and enduring bond with your child by hugging and cuddling them, making skin-to-skin contact, and figuring out your special role as a new father. Accept the pleasures and difficulties of parenthood, understanding that your love and presence have a significant influence on the growth and

the welfare of your child. Greetings from the amazing adventure of parenthood, where each encounter and moment lays the groundwork for a lifetime of love and bonding. Savor the unique link you are forming with your child during these priceless early days.

Chapter 11: Long-Term Objectives for Parenting

Being a parent is a lifelong process that changes as your child gets older. Establishing long-term parenting objectives enables you to move through this process with purpose and intention. This chapter covers developing a solid family foundation, planning for your child's future, and various parenting philosophies and techniques. You may establish a caring atmosphere that promotes your child's growth and well-being by being aware of these factors.

Philosophies and Styles of Parenting

Parenting philosophies and styles influence how you engage with your child and direct their development. Finding the ideal strategy for your family may be made easier if you are aware of the various ways.

Parenting in an authoritative manner strikes a balance between structure and warmth. In addition to being receptive and caring, authoritative parents establish clear expectations and administer regular discipline. They let kids share their ideas and emotions and promote candid conversation.

To promote comprehension and respect, you might, for instance, explain the purpose of the rule and go over the repercussions if your child disobeys it.

Authoritarian Parenting: Using stringent guidelines and high standards, authoritarian parents place a strong emphasis on compliance and discipline. This method may restrict free speech and emotional expression, even though it can foster an organized atmosphere. For example, an authoritarian parent may say, "Because I said so," without providing any additional context if your child challenges a rule.

Permissive parenting: Although they may not always enforce rules and regulations, permissive parents are kind and accommodating. They frequently give kids more freedom without establishing strict boundaries. This method can encourage freedom and creativity, but it can also cause problems with self-control and accountability. A permissive parent could, for instance, frequently let their child remain up late, putting the child's short-term needs ahead of long-term norms.

Uninvolved Parenting: Parents who are not actively engaged offer little direction, assistance, or care. Numerous things, including stress or a lack of parenting expertise, can contribute to this parenting style. Children from uninvolved homes may have trouble controlling their emotions and feeling good about themselves. Feelings of neglect may result, for example, from an absentee parent who does not participate in their child's activities or attend school functions.

Attachment parenting is a theory that places a great emphasis on developing a close emotional link with your kid through responsive feeding, co-sleeping, and babywearing. The goal of attachment parenting is to establish a stable bond that promotes emotional stability and trust. For instance, an attachment parent may calm and reassure their infant by reacting quickly to their screams.

Positive Parenting: This approach emphasizes using encouragement and praise, not punishment, to reinforce positive behavior. This strategy encourages strong relationships and self-worth. A positive parent could, for example, commend a child's efforts and provide advice on how to get better rather than reprimanding them for not finishing duties.

Future Planning: Savings, Education, and Other Aspects

Planning for your child's future entails establishing objectives and implementing doable measures to guarantee their success and well-being. Here are some important things to think about:

Education: The foundation of your child's growth is education. To determine which educational option best suits your family's requirements and values, start by looking into public, private, and homeschooling options. By helping at the school, attending parent-teacher conferences, and encouraging your child's education at home, you may remain involved in their education. The foundation of your child's growth and future achievement is education. Investigating several educational possibilities is crucial to determine which one best suits the needs and values of your family. Here are some actions to think about:

Investigate Your Options: Begin by learning about the several types of education that are accessible, including homeschooling, charter schools, private schools, and public schools. Every choice offers a unique set of benefits and things to think about. For instance, private schools might provide specialized curricula and smaller class sizes, while public schools frequently offer a variety of programs and extracurricular activities. A personalized education based on your child's interests and learning style is possible with homeschooling.

Visit Schools: Arrange to visit possible schools to meet the faculty, get a sense of the atmosphere, and discover the programs and philosophy of the institution. Talk to other parents, observe the classes, and inquire about the school's policies regarding extracurricular activities, discipline, and instruction.

Remain Active: After selecting a school, continue to be involved in your child's education. Join the parent-teacher association (PTA), volunteer at school functions, and attend parent-teacher conferences. Participating demonstrates to your child your appreciation for their education and your dedication to their achievement.

Encourage Learning at Home: Establish a peaceful study and homework area to foster a positive learning atmosphere at home. Provide a range of books and schedule family reading time to promote reading. To improve your child's learning, assist them with their assignments and projects and give them access to tools like educational websites and apps.

Promote Lifelong Learning: Encourage curiosity and discovery to cultivate a passion for learning. Bring your kids to cultural events, museums, and libraries. Urge them to look for new information and to ask questions. You may foster a lifetime love of learning in your child by encouraging a development attitude.

Savings: To secure your child's future, financial planning is crucial. Think about creating an investing plan or savings account specifically for your child's schooling and other future requirements. A 529 college savings plan, for instance, has tax benefits and can be used for approved educational costs.

To gradually accumulate a sizeable fund, begin saving early and make consistent contributions.

Open a Savings Account: Put money aside for your child's future needs, including schooling, extracurricular activities, and other long-term requirements. Seek out accounts with affordable fees and competitive interest rates. On key occasions like birthdays, encourage family members to make contributions to the account.

529 College Savings Plan: Take into account establishing a 529 college savings plan, which provides tax benefits and can be utilized for approved educational costs. Withdrawals for qualified expenses are tax-free, and contributions to a 529 plan grow tax-free. To gradually accumulate a sizeable fund, begin saving early and make consistent contributions.

Investing Accounts: Look into other investing choices, like Roth IRAs for kids or custodial accounts (UGMA/UTMA). You can invest in stocks, bonds, and mutual funds using these accounts, which could eventually yield larger returns. To find the best investment plan for your family's objectives, speak with a financial counselor.

Budgeting and Saving: Involve your child in family financial planning to help them understand the value of budgeting and saving. Make a family vacation budget, for instance, and have your kids help you keep track of your spending and save money for the trip. They learn the value of money and the significance of financial planning from this practical experience.

Emergency Fund: Set up an emergency fund to pay for unforeseen costs like house repairs or medical bills. Three to six months' worth of living expenses should be saved in a different, conveniently accessible account. Having an emergency fund gives you peace of mind and financial stability.

Health and Wellbeing: Make your child's health and well-being a top priority by arranging for routine checkups, dental procedures, and immunizations. Promote healthy behaviors including getting enough sleep, exercising frequently, and maintaining a balanced diet. The cornerstone of a healthy lifestyle is laid by teaching your child the value of wellness and self-care.

Frequent Check-Ups: To guarantee your child's health and well-being, schedule routine dental exams, medical examinations, and immunizations.

Frequent examinations support general health by identifying and addressing any health concerns early on.

Balanced Nutrition: Promote good eating practices by offering a diet full of entire grains, fruits, vegetables, lean meats, and healthy fats. Promote water as the main beverage and limit sugary snacks and drinks. To teach your child about nutrition and healthy eating, involve them in the planning and preparation of meals.

Frequent Exercise: Encourage your youngster to engage in sports, dance, or other enjoyable physical activities to foster regular physical exercise. Every day, try to get in at least 60 minutes of moderate-to-intense activity. Engaging in physical activity enhances mood, promotes general health, and aids in maintaining a healthy weight.

Adequate Sleep: Make sure your youngster receives adequate sleep by setting up a regular bedtime and making your home conducive to rest. While age-specific recommendations vary, school-aged children typically require 9–12 hours of sleep per night. For both mental and physical development, getting enough sleep is crucial.

Mental Health: Encourage open communication and create a secure environment for your child to express their emotions to support their mental health. Encourage stress-relieving and relaxation-promoting pursuits like yoga, mindfulness, and artistic hobbies. Keep an eye out for any indications of depression or anxiety, and if necessary, get professional assistance.

Life Skills: Give your child the fundamental life skills they will need far into their adult years. These abilities include effective communication, time management, problem-solving, and financial literacy. For instance, teach your child the importance of money and financial planning by having them help with budgeting and saving for a family vacation.

Financial Literacy: Instruct your youngster on budgeting, saving, and money management. Give them an allowance, for instance, and assist them in making a spending and savings plan. Talk about the idea of interest and investments, as well as the significance of saving for future objectives.

Time management: Establish a daily routine that allows time for homework, housework, extracurricular activities, and leisure to assist your child in learning time management skills. Teach kids time management skills and task prioritization by using calendars and planners. Encourage your youngster to think critically and work through issues on their own. Give them problems that are appropriate for their age and assist them in solving them. For instance, instead of giving them the solution to a challenging homework assignment, offer guided questions to help them solve it.

Good Communication: Instruct your child in good communication techniques, such as peacefully settling disagreements, active listening, and clear thinking expression. Practice these abilities by role-playing various situations and offering constructive criticism to help them get better.

Self-Care: Teach your child how to look after their physical and mental health to instill in them the value of self-care. Promote healthy behaviors including consistent exercise, a well-balanced diet, and enough sleep. Instruct them in relaxing methods and stress the value of rest periods.

Extracurricular Activities: Through extracurricular pursuits like athletics, music, art, or volunteer work, you can help your child discover their interests and skills. These pursuits foster social skills, a sense of achievement, and personal development. Encourage your child's interests and provide them with chances to hone their abilities.

Determine Interests: Take note of your child's passions and areas of interest. Find activities that suit their interests and offer chances for development, whether it's community service, athletics, music, or the arts.

Give Your Child Opportunities: Sign up for extracurricular activities that align with their interests. This can entail helping in the community, taking music lessons, painting classes, or joining a sports team. Giving your child a range of choices enables them to explore many topics and identify their areas of strength.

Encourage Commitment: By supporting your child in sticking with their chosen interests, you may teach them the importance of dedication and tenacity. Allowing kids to pursue a variety of hobbies is vital, but it also highlights the need for commitment and perseverance.

Encourage and Celebrate: Participate in your child's events, performances, and games to show your support. Honor their accomplishments and encourage them. Your support gives them more self-assurance and inspires them to keep pursuing their interests.

Balance and Well-Being: Make sure your child's schedule strikes a balance between homework, leisure time, and extracurricular activities. Don't overbook; instead, make time for leisure and family time. Burnout is avoided and general well-being is enhanced by a balanced approach.

Creating a Solid Family Basis

A solid family foundation gives your child security, encouragement, and a feeling of acceptance. The following are some strategies for creating and preserving a solid family foundation:

Encourage candid and open conversation among your family members. Establish an atmosphere where people can freely express their ideas and emotions. For instance, schedule frequent family gatherings to talk about significant issues, provide updates, and resolve any worries. Promote empathy and attentive listening to improve the bond within your family.

Quality Time: To strengthen ties and make enduring memories, spend quality time as a family. Take part in family-friendly activities like game nights, outdoor excursions, or meal preparation. Make family time a priority by scheduling frequent times to spend together and have fun.

Family customs and rituals should be established in order to foster a feeling of continuity and inclusion. These could be yearly getaways, weekly movie evenings, or holiday festivities. Family ties are strengthened and a feeling of identity is given by traditions. To make treasured memories, you may, for instance, establish a custom of baking cookies together each holiday season.

Encouragement and Support: Consistently offer each family member encouragement and support. Honor accomplishments, provide support when needed, and express gratitude for one another's work. For example, support your child at sporting events, go to school functions, and give them credit for their efforts and achievements.

Resolution of Conflicts: Handle disputes and conflicts positively. Instruct your youngster in constructive dispute resolution techniques including active listening, "I" statements, and coming up with solutions that both parties can agree on. In your relationships with your partner and other family members, set an example of polite communication and problem-solving techniques.

Shared Responsibilities: To foster cooperation and a sense of belonging, and involve everyone in household duties. Assign each family member age-appropriate duties and chores to promote cooperation and a sense of responsibility. Younger kids can help set the table, for instance, while older kids can help with yard chores or food preparation.

Emotional Support: Give your child a loving and emotionally supporting atmosphere. During trying times, pay attention to their emotional needs and provide consolation and assurance. Validate your child's emotions and encourage them to express them. For instance, listen sympathetically and provide support and direction if your child is angry about something at school.

Modeling Positive Behavior: Kids pick up skills from watching how their parents behave. In your daily contacts, set an example of virtues like compassion, respect, and fortitude. Exhibit a cheerful outlook, good communication skills, and healthy coping mechanisms. Your behavior gives your child a strong example to follow.

Community Involvement: Get involved in your neighborhood to foster a feeling of connection and belonging that extends beyond your immediate family. Build ties with friends and neighbors, volunteer together, and take part in community events. Participating in the community builds your family's support system and cultivates a sense of social responsibility.

Establishing long-term parenting objectives entails establishing a solid family foundation, anticipating your child's future, and comprehending various parenting philosophies. By adopting these components, you establish a caring atmosphere that promotes your child's development, growth, and general well-being. Your dedication to these objectives will enable you to negotiate the joys and trials of parenthood with confidence and purpose. Greetings from the fulfilling journey of parenting a contented, healthy, and well-rounded child.

Chapter 12: Materials and Assistance

Fatherhood can be a thrilling and difficult road to navigate. The experience of becoming a new father can be greatly impacted by having access to the appropriate tools and assistance. This chapter discusses helpful books, websites, and workshops for new fathers, the value of forming relationships with other fathers, and how to know when to need professional assistance.

New Fathers' books, websites, and classes

To assist new fathers in navigating the challenges of parenting, a wealth of resources are accessible. The following books, websites, and courses are highly recommended:

Books:

1. Jennifer Ash and Armin A. Brott's "The Expectant Father":
Everything from pregnancy to the first year of parenting is covered in this

extensive guide. It offers helpful guidance, consolation, and understanding of what to anticipate at every phase.

2. John Pfeiffer's "Dude, You're Gonna Be a Dad!" This book, which is written in a lighthearted and approachable manner, provides helpful pointers and counsel for expectant fathers. It addresses issues including helping your partner, getting ready for the baby, and adjusting to fatherhood in the early stages.

3. Gary Greenberg and Jeannie Hayden's book "Be Prepared: A Practical Handbook for New Dads": This book is jam-packed with useful advice, to-do lists, and images to assist new fathers in managing a variety of parenting scenarios. It includes everything from baby-proofing your house to changing diapers.

4. Scott Mactavish's book "The New Dad's Survival Guide": This manual offers simple guidance and pointers for new fathers on subjects including taking care of your child, helping your spouse, and overcoming the difficulties of parenting.

Websites:

1. Fatherly (fatherly.com): This extensive website provides tools, videos, and essays on a range of fatherhood-related topics. It addresses things like family activities, fitness and health, and parenting advice.

2. The Dad (thedad.com): This community-driven website offers dads relatable and funny content. It includes memes, movies, and articles that highlight the difficulties and rewards of fatherhood.

3. The National Fatherhood Initiative (fatherhood.org): This group provides activities and tools to help dads along the way as parents. The website offers resources, studies, and articles to support fathers in developing close bonds with their kids.

4. Dads Adventure (dadsadventure.com): This website provides information and assistance to new and expectant fathers. In addition to movies and articles, the website has a community forum where fathers may interact and exchange stories.

Courses:

1. New Dad's Boot Camp: Expectant fathers are the target audience for this interactive program. The session, which is taught by seasoned fathers, includes subjects including taking care of your child, helping your partner, and acclimating to fatherhood. It offers helpful guidance as well as a chance to voice concerns and ask questions.

2. Parenting lessons at Local Hospitals: A lot of hospitals provide pregnant patients with parenting lessons. A variety of subjects are covered in these seminars, such as breastfeeding, baby care, and preparing for childbirth. For information on available classes and timetables, contact your neighborhood hospital.

3. Online Parenting Courses: A wide range of parenting topics are covered in the many online courses that are accessible. Courses on subjects like positive parenting, sleep training, and baby care are available

on websites like Udemy, Coursera, and BabyCenter. These courses are accessible from the convenience of your home and offer flexibility.

Support Systems: Making Connections with Other Dads

Making connections with other fathers can offer helpful companionship, support, and guidance. Here are a few strategies for creating a network of support:

1. Join a Dad's Group: Regular meetings of parenting or dad's groups are held in many towns. These clubs give dads a chance to meet other dads, exchange stories, and get support. Use community centers, libraries, or internet resources like Meetup to find local groups.

2. Online Communities: Dads can interact and exchange stories in a variety of online communities and forums. There are sections specifically for fathers on websites like Reddit, BabyCenter, and The Bump. These online forums offer a forum for dads to exchange tales, ask questions, and get assistance.

3. Social media: There are pages and groups devoted to fatherhood on social media sites like Facebook and Instagram. You may interact with other fathers, take part in conversations, and obtain useful materials by joining these organizations. Seek out organizations that complement your parenting style and interests.

4. Parenting Workshops and Events: Participate in local parenting seminars, workshops, and events. These events offer a chance to network

with other parents, gain knowledge from professionals, and form support systems. For information on forthcoming events, contact the neighborhood's community centers, medical facilities, and parenting associations.

When to Get Expert Assistance

There may be occasions when professional assistance is required, even when support from books, the internet, and other fathers is priceless. Knowing when to get help from a professional is essential for your health and the health of your family.

1. Mental Health Support: It's critical to get professional assistance if you or your spouse are exhibiting signs of anxiety, depression, or other mental health conditions. Both fathers and moms may experience postpartum anxiety and depression. Persistent melancholy, anger, trouble bonding with the baby, and changes in appetite or sleep are warning signs. Seek assistance and treatment from a mental health specialist, such as a therapist or counselor.

2. Parenting Challenges: Seek advice from a pediatrician or a parenting professional if you're having particular parenting difficulties, such as trouble sleeping, eating, or dealing with behavioral disorders. These experts can offer direction, materials, and tactics to allay your worries and promote the growth of your child.

3. Relationship Support: Relationships may suffer as a result of becoming parents. Couples counseling may be helpful if you and your

partner is having problems communicating or resolving difficulties. A therapist can enhance communication, fortify your bond, and assist you in overcoming the difficulties of parenthood.

4. Health Issues: It's critical to get medical help right away if your child has health issues or developmental delays. Seeing a pediatrician on a regular basis will help you keep an eye on your child's growth and health. Do not be afraid to talk to your healthcare professional about any particular worries you may have.

Managing the parenthood path requires having access to the appropriate tools and assistance. You may guarantee a happy and satisfying experience as a new parent by reading helpful books, websites, and classes, interacting with other fathers, and knowing when to get expert assistance. Being a parent is a fulfilling journey, and you can boldly embrace its challenges and rewards with the correct support. Greetings from the amazing path of fatherhood, where every step offers fresh chances for development, love, and connection.

Conclusion

Accepting Your New Position

Being a father is an incredible adventure that is full of happiness, difficulties, and many chances for personal development. It's critical to acknowledge the significant influence you have on your child's life as well as the amazing adventures that await them as you adjust to your new role. The pleasures and difficulties of parenthood, the value of lifelong learning and development, and the necessity of commemorating your fatherhood experience will all be covered in this finale.

The Pleasures and Difficulties of Parenting

The special mix of happiness and difficulties that come with becoming a father molds your experience and deepens your relationship with your child. Here are a few important factors to think about:

The pleasures:

1. Unconditional affection: Feeling your child's unconditional affection is one of the greatest pleasures of parenting. You will have an intense and enduring bond with your child that gets stronger every day from the first time you hold them. There is a great deal of joy and happiness in this relationship.

2. Milestones and Achievements: It is immensely satisfying to see your child accomplish new abilities and attain milestones. Every significant event, such as their first grin, first steps, or first words, demonstrates their development and progress. A sense of pride and treasured memories are produced when people celebrate these occasions together.

3. Shared Experiences: Being a father presents a wealth of chances to spend time with your child. These times of enjoyment and connection, whether it be through games, bedtime stories, family vacations, or trying new things, deepen your relationship and provide enduring memories.

4. Personal Development: Being a father forces you to change and develop as a person. It promotes the growth of resilience, empathy, and patience. You'll find new qualities and capacities in yourself as you work through the highs and lows of parenthood.

The Difficulties:

1. Balancing Responsibilities: Juggling the many duties that accompany parenthood is one of the main difficulties of fatherhood. It might be difficult to balance childcare, housework, and employment. Finding a balance that enables you to complete your obligations and still find time for rest and self-care is crucial.

2. Sleep Deprivation: As you become used to your baby's sleep routine, the first few months of parenthood are frequently accompanied by sleep deprivation. Your mood and energy levels might be affected by sleep deprivation. This difficulty can be lessened by figuring out how to divide up the nocturnal chores with your spouse and get your infant to follow a regular sleep schedule.

3. Emotional Strain: Managing the demands and uncertainties of parenthood can cause emotional strain for fathers. Feeling overburdened, nervous, or uncertain occasionally is normal. You can get important advice and comfort by asking your partner, family, friends, or a therapist for help.

4. Adapting to Change: Being a parent is an ongoing process of adaptation and change. Your parenting style will need to change as your child gets older since their demands and actions will change as well. You can handle these changes with confidence if you embrace flexibility and are receptive to new information.

Ongoing Education and Development

Being a father is a lifelong learning and development process. By adopting this perspective, you may become the greatest father you can be and provide your child with a loving and supportive atmosphere. Here are a few strategies to encourage lifelong learning and development:

1. Remain Informed: Become knowledgeable about parenting techniques, child growth, and health and wellness. To keep up with the most recent findings and recommended procedures, read books, go to workshops, and visit reliable websites. Possessing knowledge enables you to make wise choices and give your child the best care possible.

2. Think and Adjust: Give your parenting experiences some thought and pinpoint areas that need work. Be receptive to criticism from other parents, your family, and your partner. Adapt your strategy to your child's needs and the dynamics of your family. As a parent, you develop by constant introspection and adjustment.

3. Seek Support: When assistance is required, don't be afraid to ask for it. Participate in online networks, interact with other fathers, and join parenting groups. Learning from others and exchanging experiences can yield insightful information and motivation. Keep in mind that you are not traveling alone and that asking for help is a show of strength.

4. Accept Challenges: See obstacles as chances for development. As a parent, every challenge presents an opportunity to grow resilient and acquire new abilities. Take on obstacles with a good outlook and an open mind. Overcoming obstacles with your child improves character development and your relationship.

5. Celebrate Your Progress: Give yourself credit for your fatherhood accomplishments. Acknowledge the minor triumphs and significant achievements you make along the journey. Honoring your development and achievements reaffirms your resolve to be a devoted and caring father.

Honoring Your Fatherhood Journey

Being a father is a journey to be honored. Enjoy the good times, think back on the difficulties you've faced, and be proud of the affection and attention you give your child. Here are some ideas for commemorating your fatherhood journey:

1. Establish Traditions: Start family customs that honor your fatherhood. These customs, whether they be a monthly "dad and me" day, an annual family vacation, or a special Father's Day activity, help you and your child form lasting memories.

2. Record Memories: Use journals, photographs, and films to preserve the unique experiences of parenting. You can reflect on the voyage and revisit the treasured memories by recording your experiences. Make a digital album or scrapbook to keep these memories for years to come.

3. Tell Stories: Tell others about your experiences as a father. Sharing your experiences can encourage and support other fathers, whether you do it on social media, via a blog, or in discussions with friends and family. It also gives you a chance to take stock of your development and acknowledge your successes.

4. Express Gratitude: Give thanks for the blessings and pleasures of parenting some time. Think back on the times when you feel content and happy. Gratitude increases your appreciation for the adventure and cultivates a good outlook.

5. Make Self-Care a Priority: Taking care of yourself is just as important as celebrating your experience as a father. Make self-care a

priority by doing things that make you happy and calm you down. Your well-being and capacity to be a present and involved father depend on taking care of yourself, whether that means exercising, taking up a hobby, or hanging out with friends.

Accepting your new role as a father is a journey that is full of happiness, difficulties, and ongoing development. You may foster a loving and supportive environment for your family by acknowledging the significant influence you have on your child's life and remaining dedicated to learning, growing, and appreciating your journey. Being a father is an incredible journey, and your presence, commitment, and love make all the difference. Welcome to the amazing adventure of parenthood, where you have the chance to make enduring memories and develop a close, loving relationship with your kid at every turn. Congratulations on accepting this new position and appreciating its difficulties and rewards.

With appreciation,
Dr. Elvira S. Graves

Kindly Drop a positive review for this book online, if you got value from it.
Thank you.
You can also check out my other books through this link…
https://www.amazon.com/author/elvygraves